MW00837106

Sweetie

A Story About a Girl Who Was Diagnosed with Type 1 Diabetes

LAURA SELF

Copyright © 2022 Laura Self
All rights reserved
First Edition

Fulton Books, Inc.
Meadville, PA

Published by Fulton Books 2022

ISBN 978-1-63710-911-3 (hardcover)
ISBN 978-1-63710-910-6 (digital)

Printed in the United States of America

To Hannah, my very own Sweetie

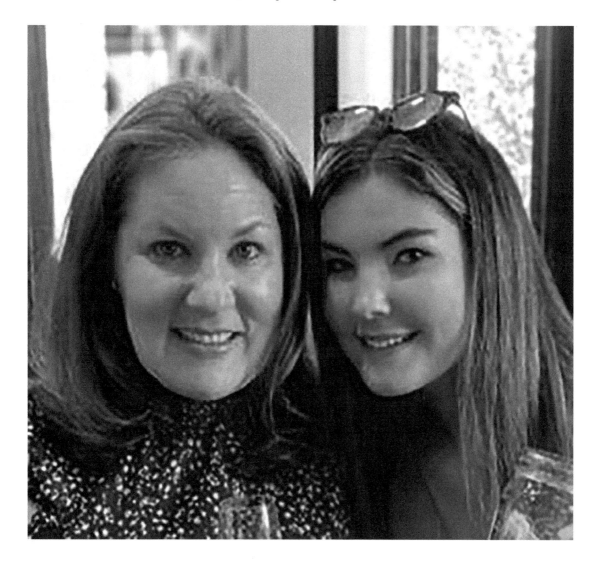

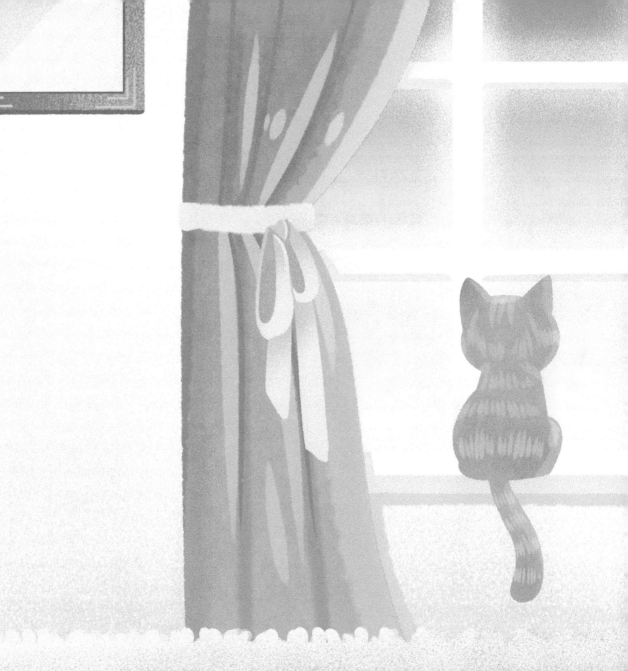

Sweetie was a little girl,
As sweet as she could be.

Sweetie loved her dolls, her cat,
Her friends, and family.

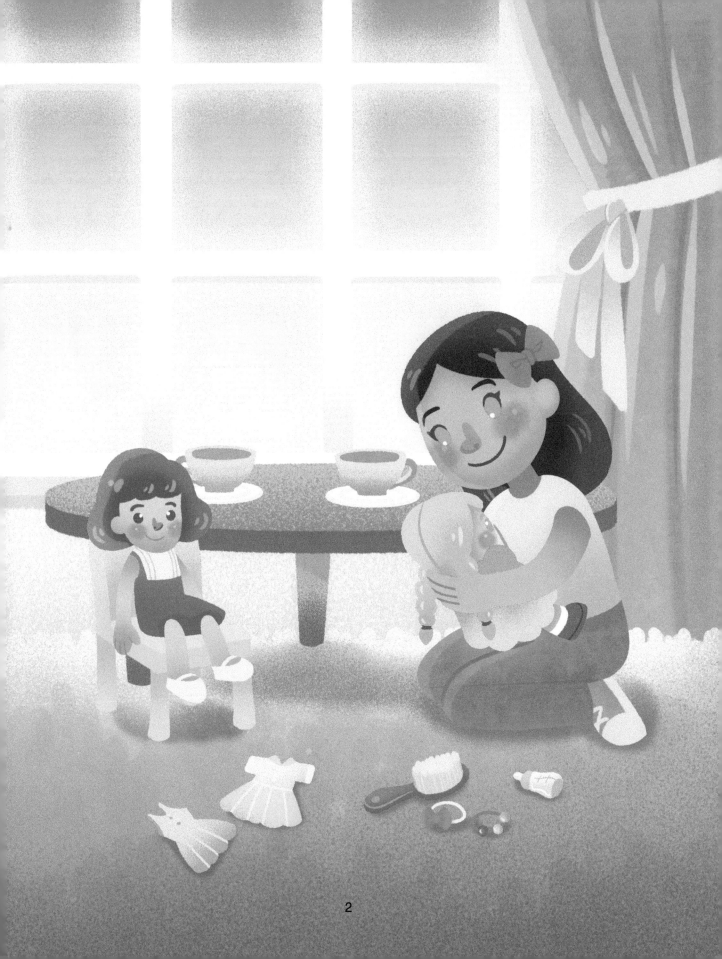

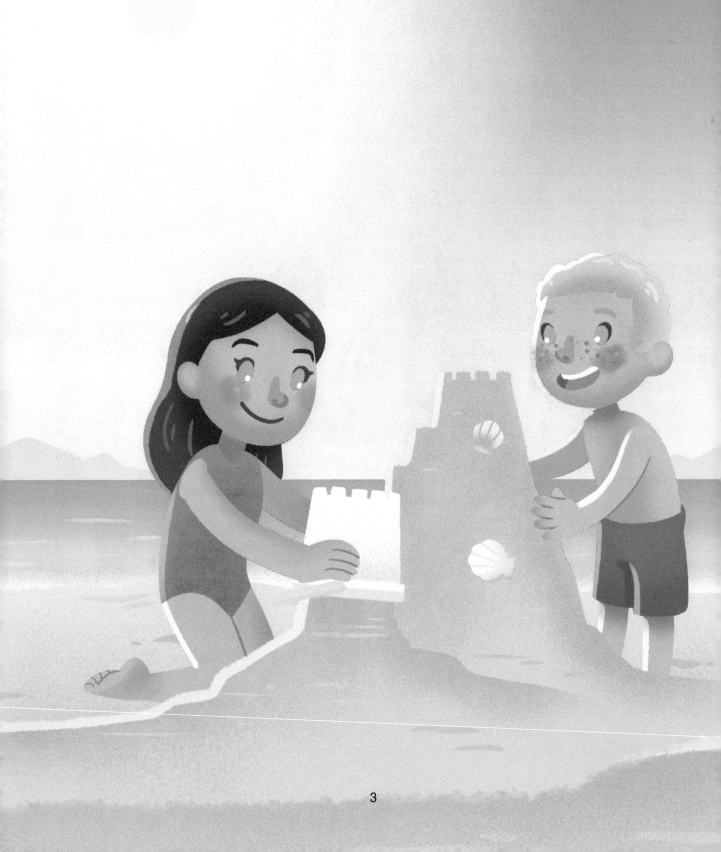

She danced, she played, she loved the beach,
All her dreams were in her reach.

Sweetie's life was going swell,
'Til she stopped feeling well.

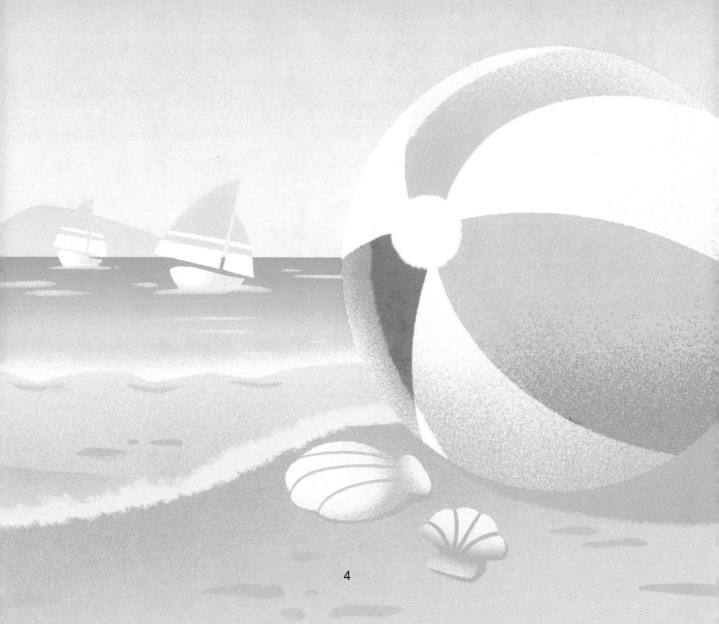

Sweetie started to feel crummy,
Her head hurt, her eyes, and her tummy.

She always thirsted for some water,
Her parents were worried about their daughter.

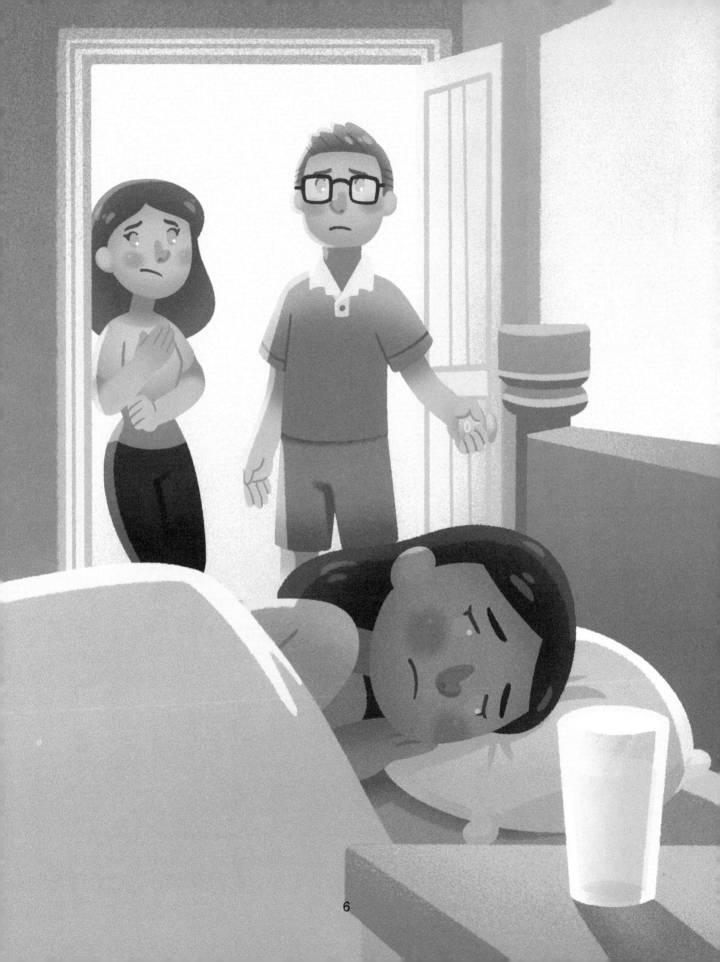

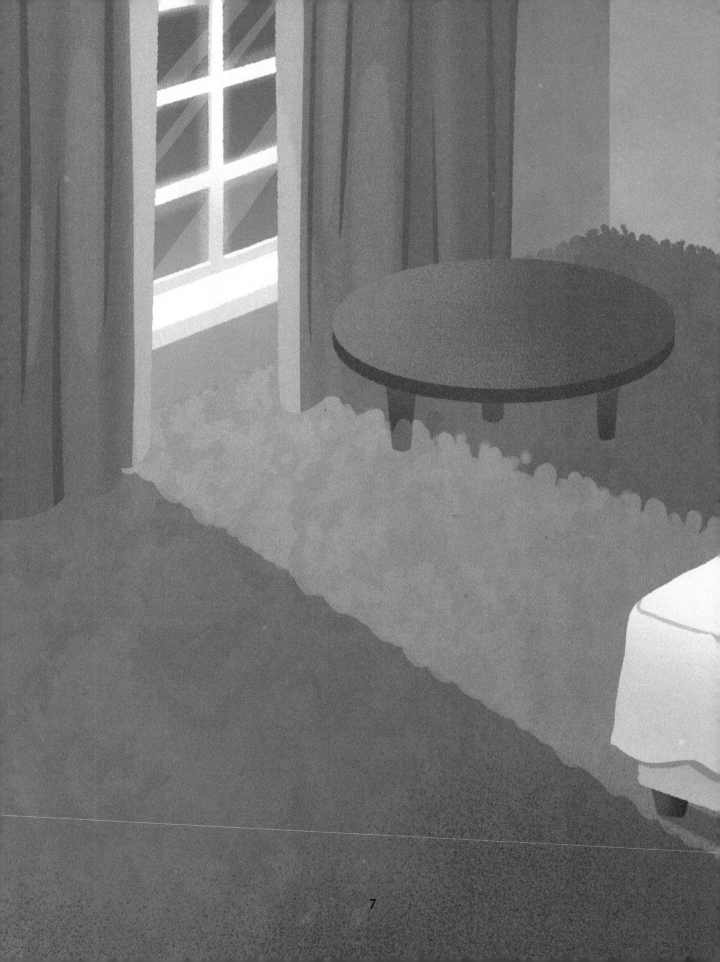

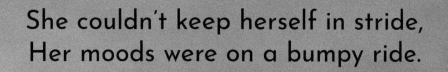

She couldn't keep herself in stride,
Her moods were on a bumpy ride.

She slept and slept and still felt slow,
What was changing? She didn't know.

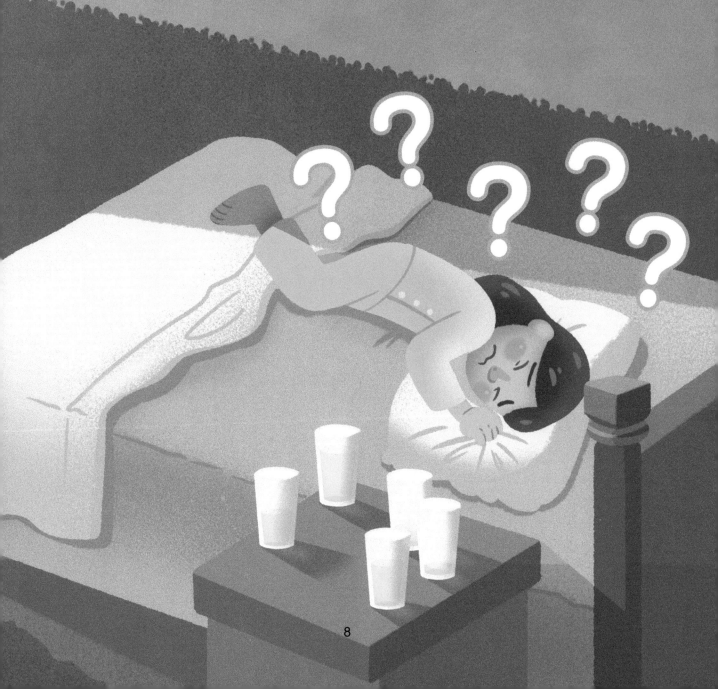

8

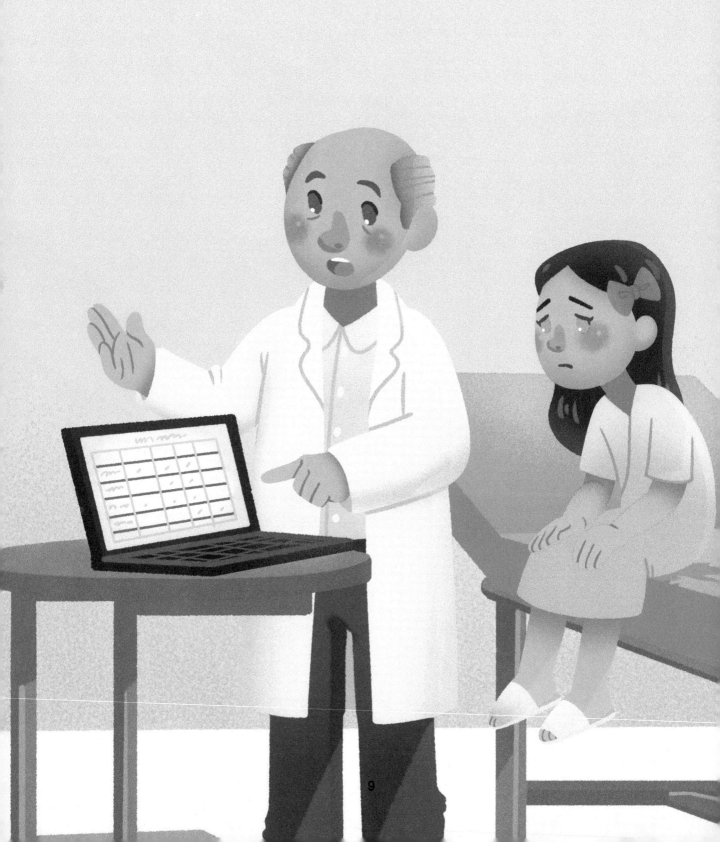

Her pancreas, the doctors say,
Had stopped its work upon that day.

No longer would her body host,
The medicine she needed most.

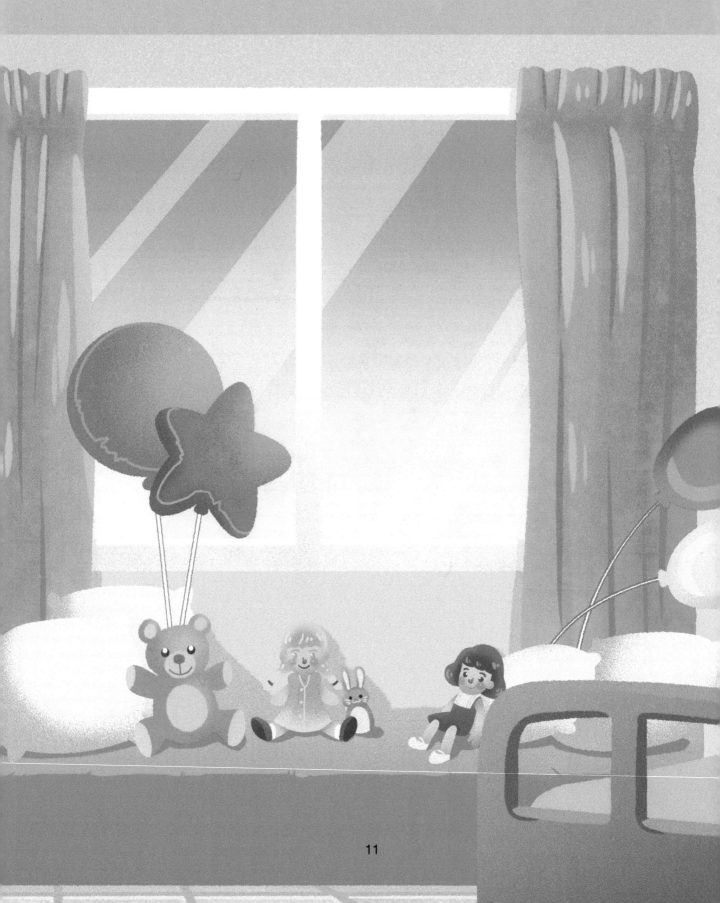

She had to have another way,
To get some insulin and save the day.

In the hospital is where they taught Sweetie,
All about type 1 diabetes.

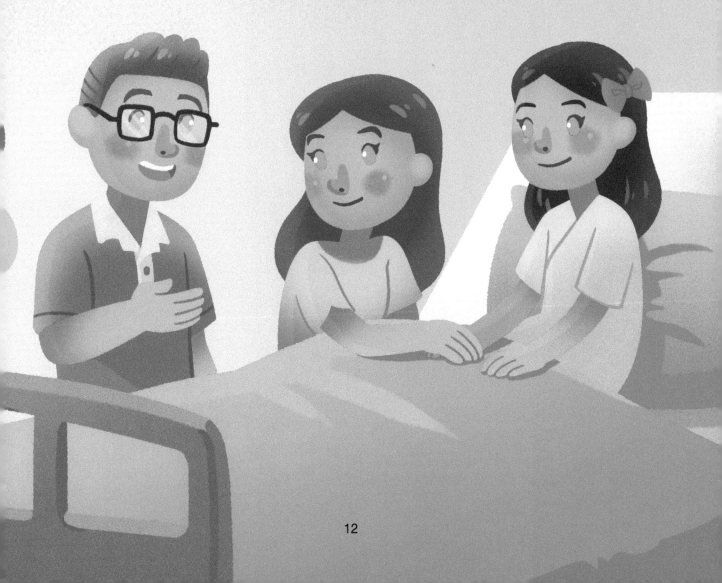

She learned the things to know,
For her to live and love and grow.

Sweetie began to count her food,
Feeling better changed her mood!

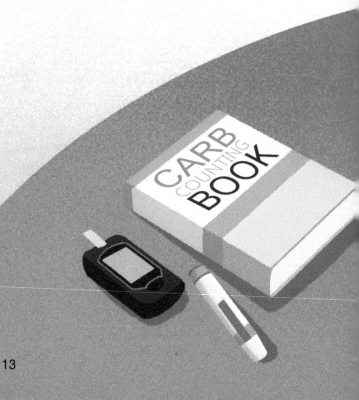

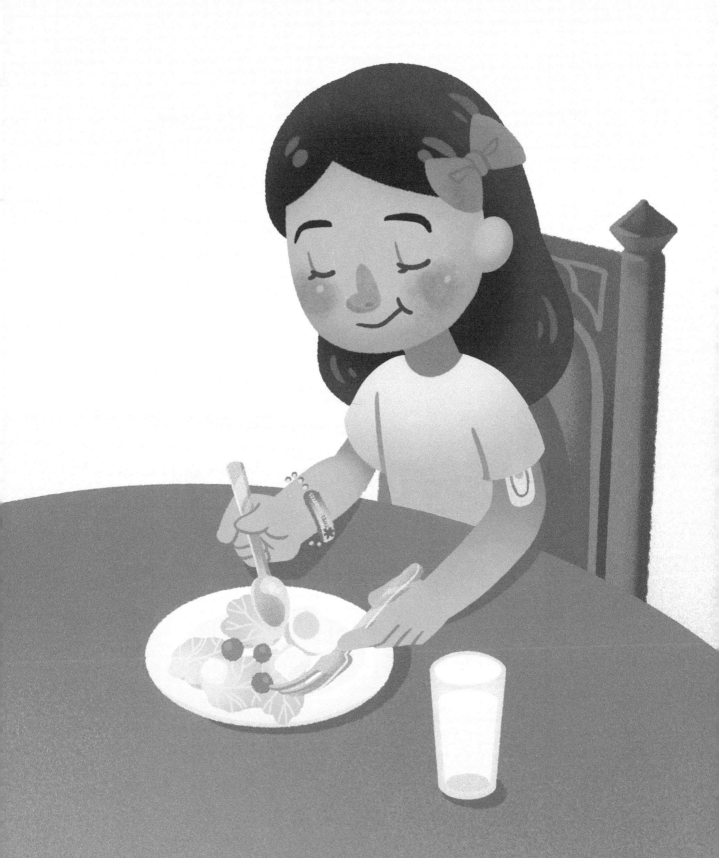

She learned about her highs and lows,
And how to make her insulin pump go.

She even got a CGM[1],
To show her how her sugars trend.

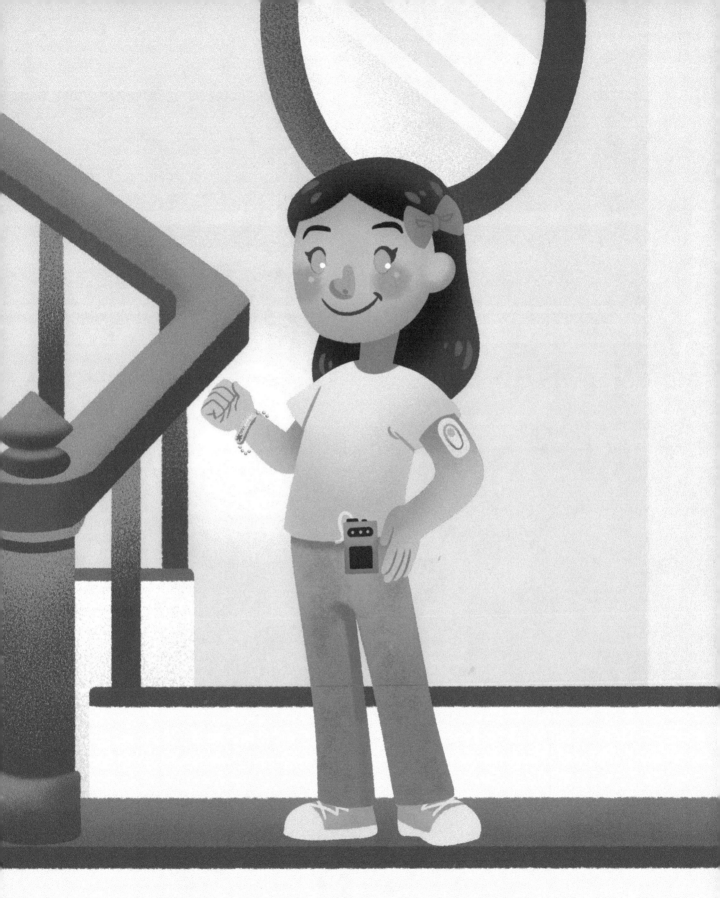

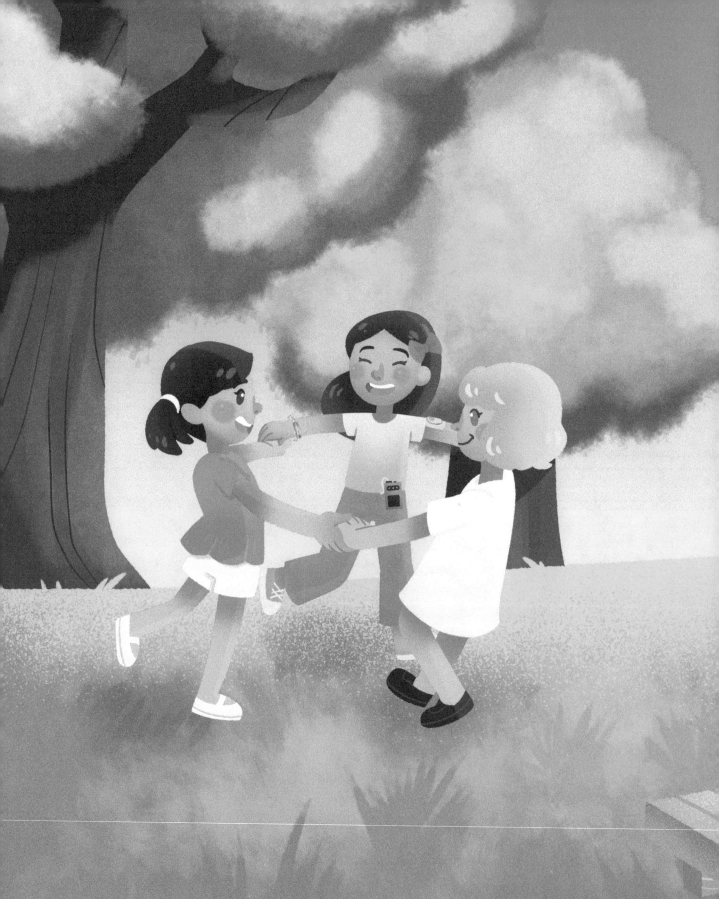

Whenever she needed a little snack,
She was prepared; she didn't lack.

Sweetie's friends stayed by her side,
And helped her when she really tried.

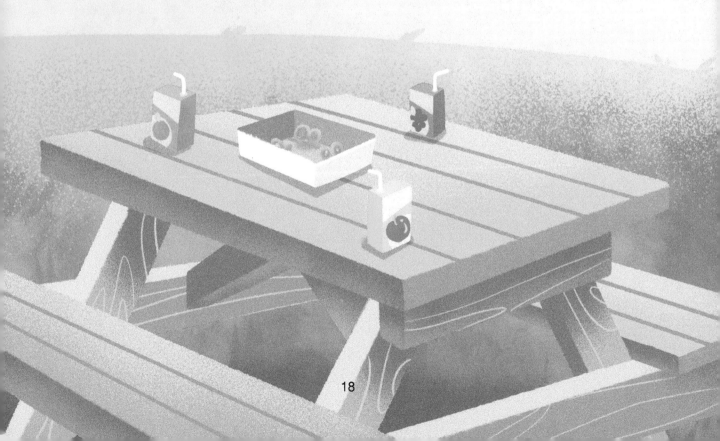

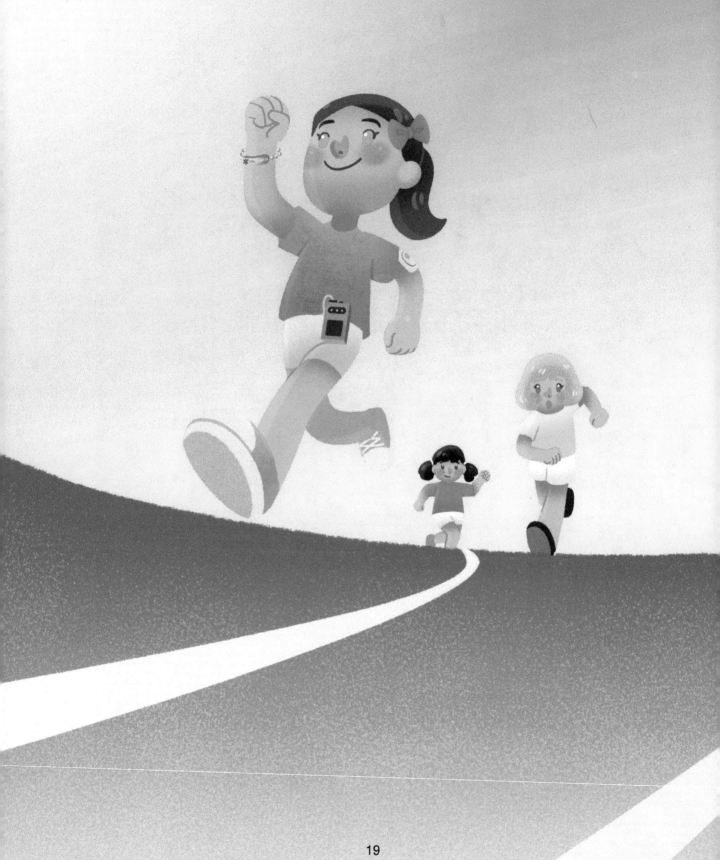

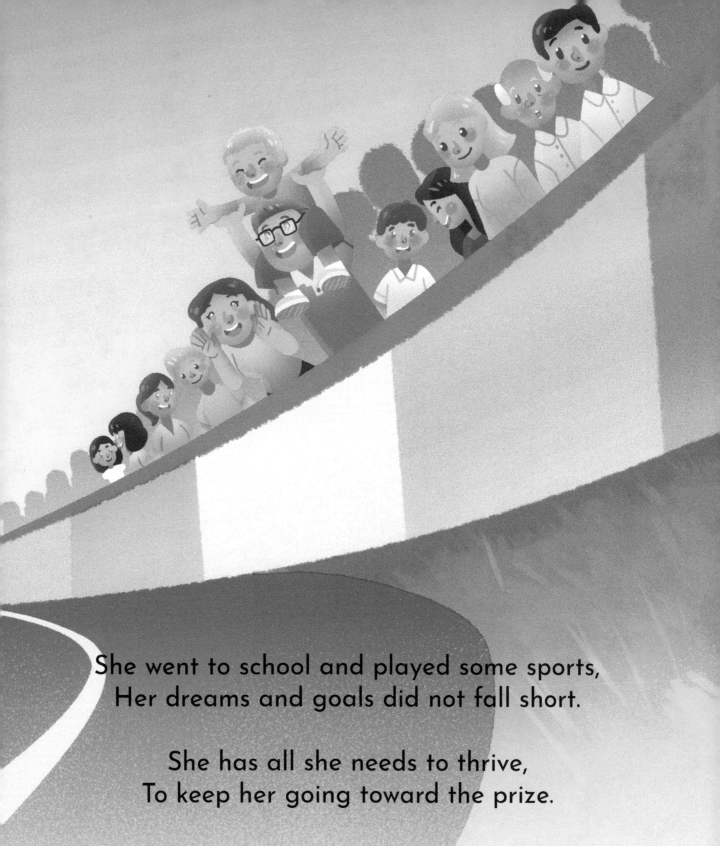

She went to school and played some sports,
Her dreams and goals did not fall short.

She has all she needs to thrive,
To keep her going toward the prize.

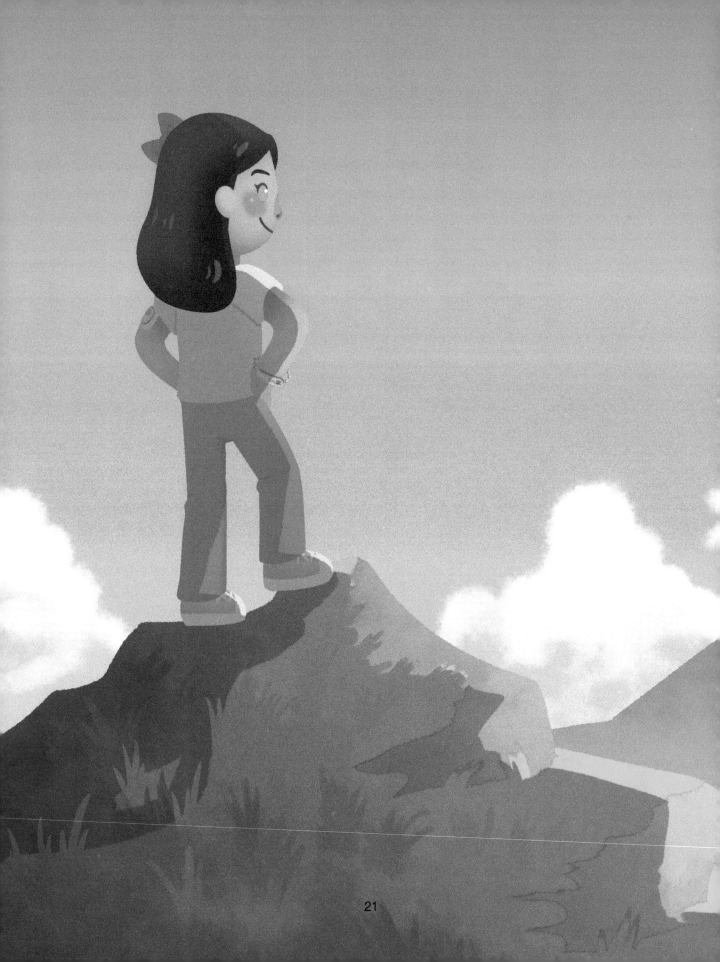

Sweetie's still the girl she always was,
She's smiley, happy, and full of love.

She learned to be so brave and strong,
Overcoming all that came along.

And on her birthday every year,
There are so many things to cheer.

Celebrating all that she's been through,
She has her cake and eats it too!

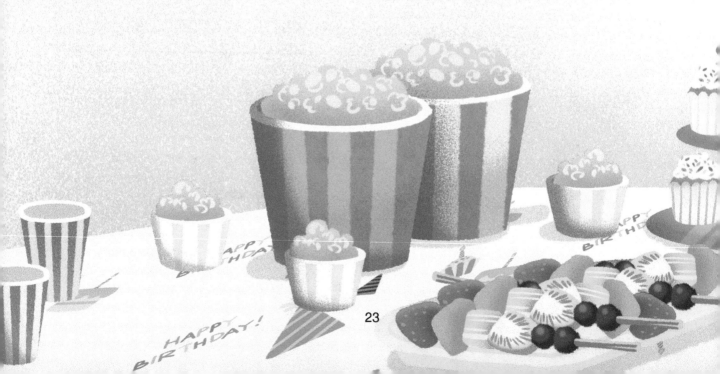

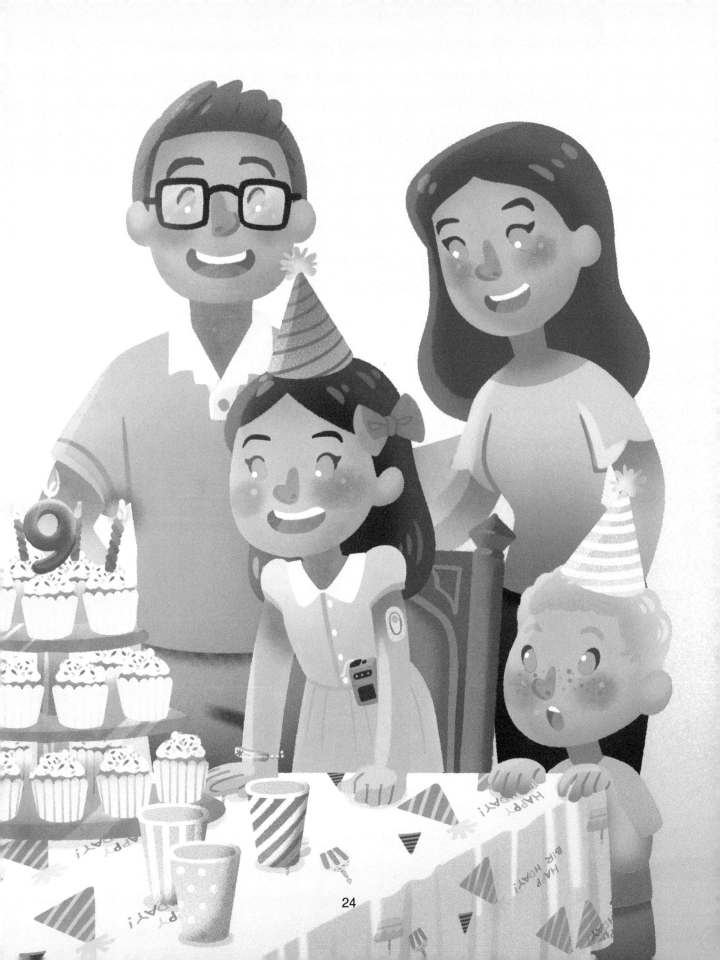

Warning signs of Type One Diabetes

Warning signs of T1D often appear suddenly and may include:

- Drowsiness or lethargy
- Extreme thirst
- Frequent urination
- Fruity odor on the breath
- Increased appetite
- Heavy or labored breathing
- Sudden weight loss
- Sudden vision changes
- Sugar in the urine
- Stupor or unconsciousness[2]

---

[2] JDRF, 2021. www.jdrf.org.

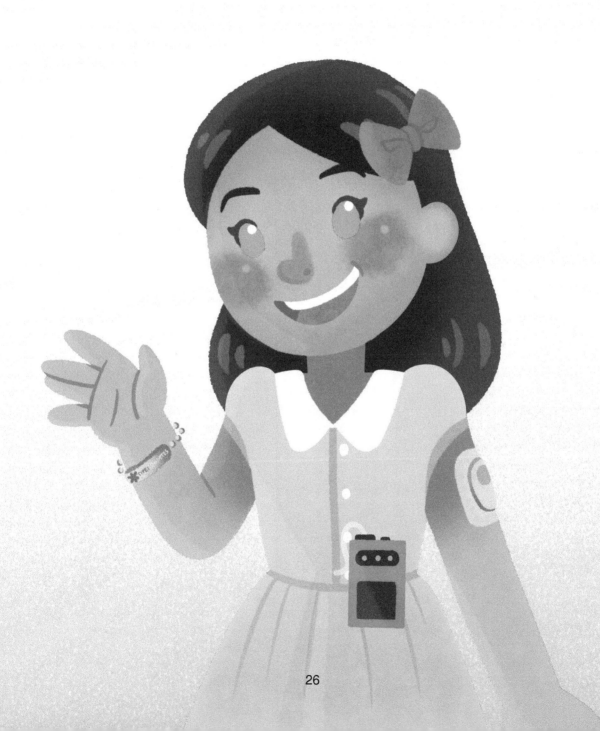

About the Author

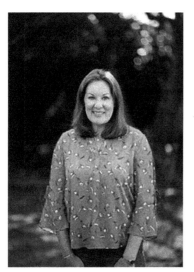 Laura Self is a Montessori teacher who works with preschoolers and loves to use books as a teaching tool for helping young children understand difficult concepts. As a mom, Laura's very own "Sweetie," Hannah, was diagnosed with type 1 diabetes when she was eight years old. *Sweetie* is the book she wished she had in the hospital when Hannah was first diagnosed. She hopes it will bring encouragement and hope to others who know and love someone with type 1 diabetes or who live with the disease themselves. Laura lives in South Carolina with her husband and their two children. Laura is the owner, director, and lead teacher at Journey Montessori Academy in Charlotte, North Carolina.

CPSIA information can be obtained
at www.ICGtesting.com
Printed in the USA
BVHW022100010522
635336BV00007B/5